CU00691370

KETO
COOKBOOK

Easy and Tasty Recipes for Weight Loss and Healthy Eating

JILL FOX

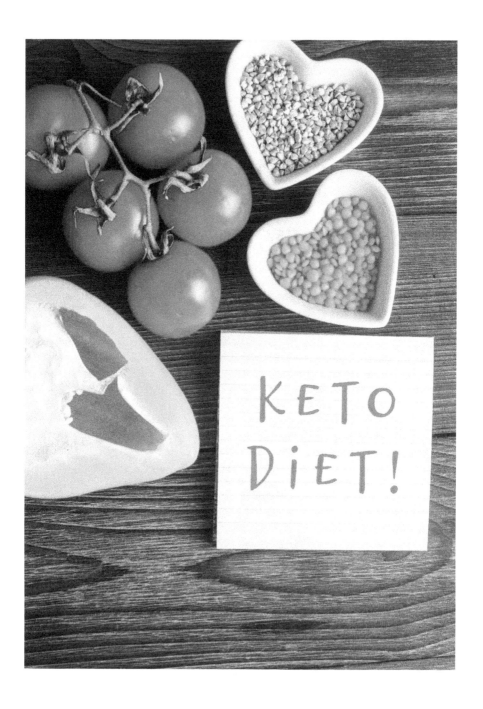

Table of Contents

Sommario

Introduction

The ketogenic diet, or keto diet, is a low carb, high-fat diet that gives many health benefits.

Many studies show that this sort of diet can assist you to reduce and improve your health.

Ketogenic diets may even have benefits against diabetes, cancer, epilepsy, and Alzheimer's disease.

What is a ketogenic diet?

The ketogenic diet is low carb, a high-fat diet that shares many similarities with the Atkins and low carb diets.

It involves drastically reducing carbohydrate intake and replacing it with fat. This reduction in carbs puts your body into a metabolic state called ketosis.

When this happens, your body becomes incredibly efficient at burning fat for energy. It also turns fat into ketones within the liver, which may supply energy for the brain

Ketogenic diets can cause significant reductions in blood glucose and insulin levels. This, alongside the increased ketones, has some health benefits.

Different types of ketogenic diets

There are several versions of the ketogenic diet, including:

The standard ketogenic diet (SKD): This is often a low carb, moderate protein, and high-fat diet. It typically contains 70% fat, 20% protein, and only 10% carbs (9Trusted Source).

The cyclical ketogenic diet (CKD): This diet involves periods of upper carb refeeds, like 5 ketogenic days followed by 2 high carb days.

The targeted ketogenic diet (TKD): This diet allows you to feature carbs around workouts.

High protein ketogenic diet: this is often almost like a typical ketogenic diet, but includes more protein. The ratio is usually 60% fat, 35% protein, and 5% carbs.

However, only the quality and high protein ketogenic diets are studied extensively. Cyclical or targeted ketogenic diets are more advanced methods and are primarily employed by bodybuilders or athletes.

What is ketosis?

Ketosis may be a metabolic state during which your body uses fat for fuel rather than carbs.
It occurs once you significantly reduce your consumption of carbohydrates, limiting your body's supply of glucose (sugar), which is that the main source of energy for the cells.
Following a ketogenic diet is that the best thanks to entering ketosis. Generally, this involves limiting carb consumption to around 20 to 50 grams per day and filling abreast of fats, like meat, fish, eggs, nuts, and healthy oils
It's also important to moderate your protein consumption, this is often because protein can be converted into glucose if consumed in high amounts, which can slow your transition into ketosis
Practicing intermittent fasting could also assist you to enter ketosis faster. There are many various sorts of intermittent fasting, but the foremost common method involves limiting food intake to around 8 hours per day and fasting for the remaining 16 hours
Blood, urine, and breath tests are available, which may help determine whether you've entered ketosis by measuring the number of ketones produced by your body.

Certain symptoms can also indicate that you've entered ketosis, including increased thirst, dry mouth, frequent urination, and decreased hunger or appetite

Ketogenic diets can help you lose weight

A ketogenic diet is also an effective solution for losing weight and decreasing risk factors for disease.
Research has shown that the ketogenic diet can be very effective for weight loss as a low-fat diet.
What's more, the diet is so rich that you can lose weight without needing to count calories or track your food intake.
An analysis of 13 studies revealed that following a low-carb ketogenic diet was slightly superior for long-term weight loss compared to a low-fat diet.
It also led to a reduction in diastolic blood pressure and triglyceride levels.

Other health benefits of keto

- The ketogenic diet originated as a method of treating neurological diseases such as epilepsy.
- Studies have now shown that this diet may have benefits for a wide variety of different health conditions:

- Heart disease. The ketogenic diet can help improve risk factors such as body fat, HDL (good) cholesterol levels, blood pressure, and blood sugar.

- Cancer. Diet is currently being explored as an adjunct treatment for cancer because it may help slow tumor growth.

- Alzheimer's disease. The keto diet may help reduce the symptoms of Alzheimer's disease and slow its progression.

- Epilepsy. Research has shown that the ketogenic diet can cause significant reductions in seizures in epileptic children.

- Parkinson's disease. Although more research is needed, one study found that the diet helped improve symptoms of Parkinson's disease.

- Polycystic ovary syndrome. The ketogenic diet may help reduce insulin levels, which may play a key role in polycystic ovary syndrome.

- Brain injury. Some research suggests that the diet may improve the outcomes of traumatic brain injuries.

However, keep in mind that research in many of these areas is far from conclusive.

Foods to avoid

Any food high in carbohydrates should be reduced.
Here is a list of foods that should be reduced or eliminated on a ketogenic diet:

sugary foods: soda, juice, smoothies, cake, ice cream, candy, etc.
grains or starches: wheat products, rice, pasta, cereals, etc.
fruits: all fruits, except small portions of berries such as strawberries
beans or legumes: peas, beans, lentils, chickpeas, etc.
root and tuber vegetables: potatoes, sweet potatoes, carrots, parsnips, etc.

low-fat or diet products: low-fat mayonnaise, salad dressings, and condiments
some condiments or sauces: barbecue sauce, honey mustard, teriyaki sauce, ketchup, etc.
unhealthy fats: processed vegetable oils, mayonnaise, etc.
alcohol: beer, wine, liquor, mixed drinks
sugar-free diet foods: sugar-free candy, syrups, puddings, sweeteners, desserts, etc.

Foods to eat

You should focus most of your meals on these foods:

meat: red meat, steak, ham, sausage, bacon, chicken, and turkey
fatty fish: salmon, trout, tuna, and mackerel
eggs: whole pastured eggs or omega-3s
butter and cream: grass-fed butter and heavy cream
cheese: non-processed cheeses such as cheddar, goat, cream, blue, or mozzarella cheese
nuts and seeds: almonds, walnuts, flaxseeds, pumpkin seeds, chia seeds, etc.
healthy oils: extra virgin olive oil, coconut oil, and avocado oil
avocado: whole avocado or freshly made guacamole
low carb vegetables: green vegetables, tomatoes, onions, peppers, etc.
seasonings: salt, pepper, herbs, and spices
It's best to base your diet primarily on whole, single-ingredient foods. Here's a list of 44 healthy low-carb foods.

Healthy keto snacks

In case you get the urge to eat between meals, here are some healthy, keto-approved snacks:

fatty meat or fish
cheese
a handful of nuts or seeds
keto sushi bites
olives
one or two hard-boiled or deviled eggs
keto-friendly snack bars
90 percent dark chocolate
whole Greek yogurt mixed with nut butter and cocoa powder
peppers and guacamole
strawberries and plain cottage cheese
celery with salsa and guacamole
beef jerky
smaller portions of leftover meals
fat bombs

Keto tips and tricks

Although starting the ketogenic diet can be difficult, there are several tips and tricks you can use to make it easier.

Start by familiarizing yourself with food labels and checking the grams of fat, carbohydrates, and fiber to determine how your favorite foods can fit into your diet.
Planning your meals can also be beneficial and can help you save extra time during the week.

Tips for eating out on a ketogenic diet

Many restaurant meals can be made keto-friendly.

Most restaurants offer some type of meat or fish dish. Order this food and replace any high-carb food with extra vegetables.

Egg meals are also a good option, such as an omelet or eggs and bacon.

Another favorite meal is burgers without a bun. You could also replace the fries with veggies. Add extra avocado, cheese, bacon, or eggs.

In Mexican restaurants, you can enjoy any type of meat with extra cheese, guacamole, salsa, and sour cream.

For dessert, ask for a tray of mixed cheeses or berries with cream.

At least, in the beginning, it's crucial to eat until you're full and avoid cutting calories too much. Usually, a ketogenic diet involves weight loss without intentional calorie restriction.

In this Keto cookbook, you can organize your Keto diet with the different dishes you'll find for meals throughout the day. Enjoy!

Breakfast

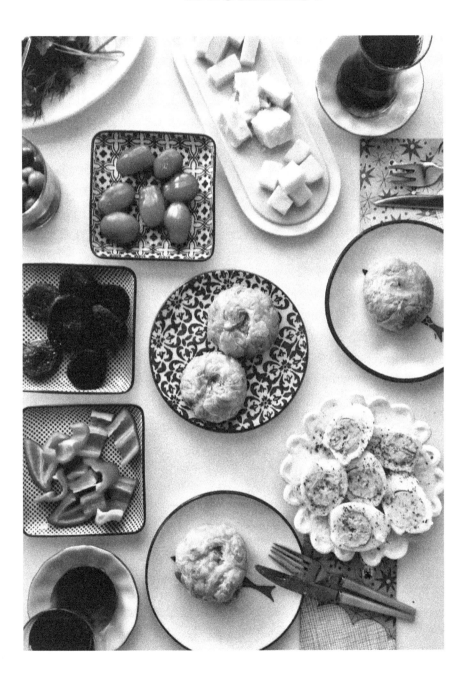

Goat Cheese Frittata

Preparation Time: 15 minutes
Cooking Time: 15 minutes
Servings: 4

Ingredients:
tbsp. avocado oil for frying
oz. (56 g) bacon slices, chopped
1 red bell pepper
small yellow onion, chopped
scallions, chopped
1 tbsp. chopped fresh chives
Salt and black pepper to taste
8 eggs, beaten
1 tbsp. unsweetened almond milk
1 tbsp. chopped fresh parsley
3 1/2 oz. (100 g) goat cheese, divided 3/4 oz. (20 g) grated Parmesan cheese

Directions:
Let the oven preheat to 350°F/175°C. Heat the avocado oil in a medium cast-iron pan and cook the bacon for 5 minutes or golden brown. Stir in the bell pepper, onion, scallions, and chives. Cook for 3 to 4 minutes or until the vegetables soften. Season with salt and black pepper. In a bowl or container, the eggs must be beaten with the almond milk and parsley. Pour the mixture over the vegetables, stirring to spread out nicely. Share half of the goat cheese on top. Once the eggs start to set, divide the remaining goat cheese on top, season with salt, black pepper, and place the pan in the oven—Bake for 5 to 6 minutes or until the eggs set all around.
Take out the pan, scatter the Parmesan cheese on top, slice, and serve warm.

Nutrition:
Calories: 412; Fat: 15.4g; Fiber: 11.2g; Carbohydrates: 4.9 g; Protein: 10.5g

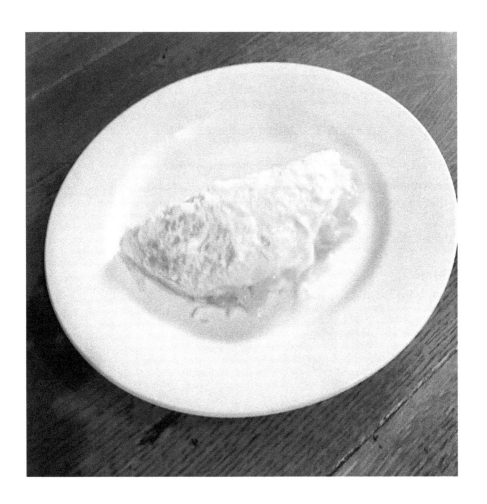

Easy Buttery Oatmeal

Preparation time: 10 minutes
Cooking time: 3 hours
Servings: 2

Ingredients:
Cooking spray
2 cups coconut milk
1 cup old fashioned oats
1 pear, cubed
1 apple, cored and cubed 2 tablespoons butter, melted

Directions:
Grease your slow cooker with the cooking spray, add the milk, oats and the other ingredients, toss, put the lid on and cook on High for 3 hours.
Divide the mix into bowls and serve for breakfast.

Nutrition:
Calories 1002,
Fat 74,
Fiber 18,
Carbs 93,
Protein 16.2

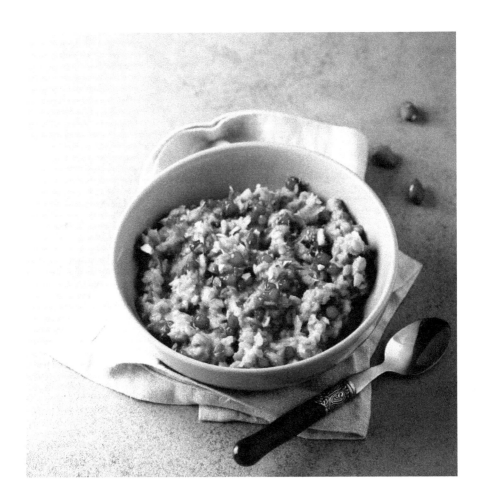

Fluffy Chocolate Pancakes

Preparation Time: 15 minutes
Cooking Time: 12 minutes
Servings: 4

Ingredients:
 2 cups (250 g) almond flour
2 tsp. baking powder
2 tbsp... Erythritol
3/4 tsp. salt
2 eggs
1/3 cups (320 ml) almond milk
tbsp. butter + more for fryingTopping:
2 tbsp. unsweetened chocolate buttons
Sugar-free maple syrup 4 tbsp. semi-salted butter

Directions:

In a bowl or container, mix the almond flour, baking powder, Erythritol, and salt. Whisk the eggs, almond milk, and butter in another bowl. Combine in the dry ingredients and mix well. Melt about 1 1/2 tablespoon of butter in a non-stick skillet, pour in portions of the batter to make small circles, about two pieces per batch (approximately 1/4 cup of batter each). Sprinkle some chocolate buttons on top and cook for 1 to 2 minutes or until set beneath. Turn the pancakes and cook for one more minute or until set. Remove the pancakes onto a plate and make more with the remaining ingredients. Work with more butter and reduce the heat as needed to prevent sticking and burning. Drizzle the pancakes with some maple syrup, top with more butter (as desired), and enjoy!

Nutrition:
Calories: 384
Fat: 12.9g
Fiber: 5.4g
Carbohydrates: 7.5 g

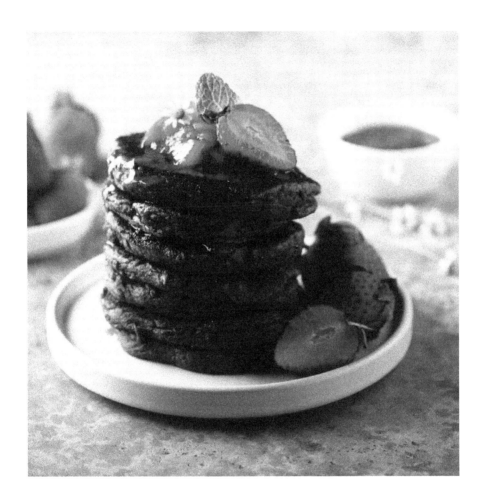

Mushroom and Bell Pepper Omelet

Preparation time: 5 minutes
Cooking time: 5 minutes
Servings: 4

Ingredients:
2 tablespoons olive oil
cup Chanterelle mushrooms, chopped
bell peppers, chopped
1 white onion, chopped
6 eggs

Directions:
Heat the olive oil in a nonstick skillet over moderate heat. Now, cook the mushrooms, peppers, and onion until they have softened.
In a mixing bowl, whisk the eggs until frothy. Add the eggs to the skillet, reduce the heat to medium-low, and cook approximately 5 minutes until the center starts to look dry. Do not overcook.
Taste and season with salt to taste. Bon appétit!

Nutrition:
calories: 240
fat: 17.5g
protein: 12.3g
carbs: 6.1g
net carbs: 4.3g
fiber: 1.8g

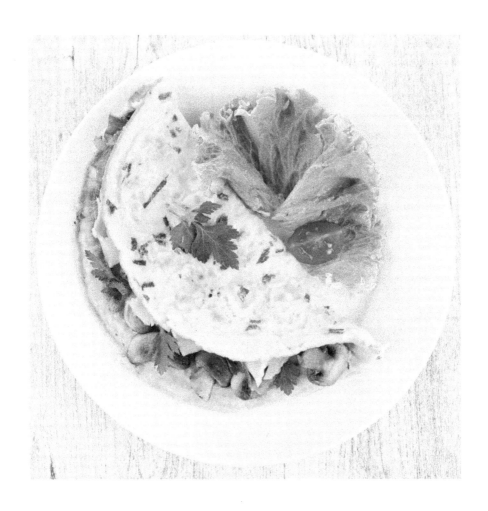

Mozzarella Italian Peppers

Preparation time: 7 minutes
Cooking time: 13 minutes
Servings: 5

Ingredients:
4 tablespoons canola oil
1 yellow onion, sliced
1⅓ pounds (605 g) Italian peppers, deveined and sliced
teaspoon Italian seasoning mix
Sea salt and cayenne pepper, to season

Directions:
balls buffalo Mozzarella, drained and halved
Heat the canola oil in a saucepan over a medium-low flame. Now, sauté the onion until just tender and translucent.
Add in the peppers and spices. Cook for about 13 minutes, adding a splash of water to deglaze the pan.
Divide between serving plates; top with cheese and serve immediately. Enjoy!

Nutrition:
calories: 175
fat: 11.0g
protein: 10.4g
carbs: 7.0g
net carbs: 5.1g
fiber: 1.9g

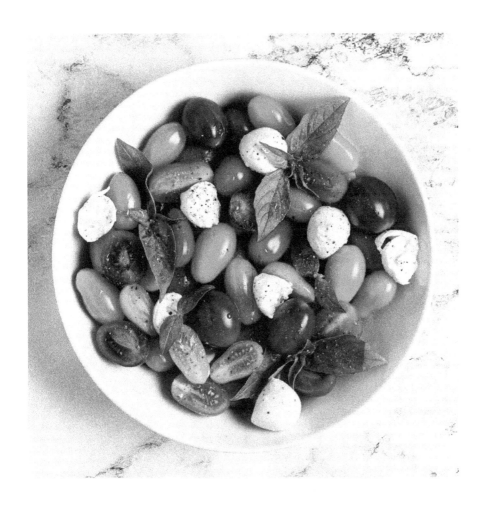

Chicken

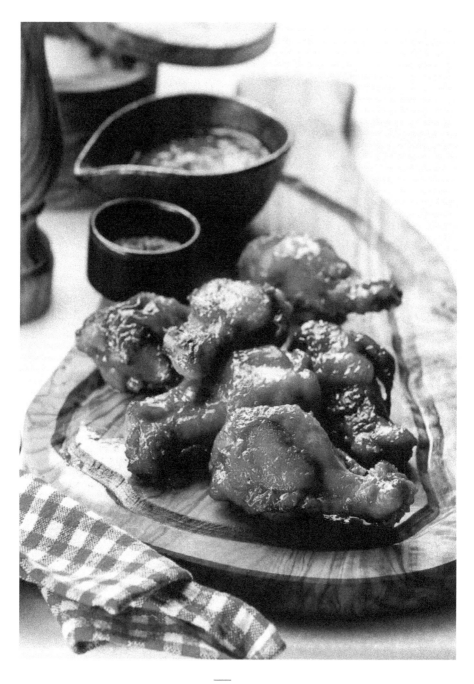

Spiced Duck Goulash

Preparation time: 15 minutes
Cooking time: 5 minutes
Servings: 2

Ingredients:
2 (1-ounce / 28-g) slices bacon, chopped
½ pound (227 g) duck legs, skinless and boneless
2 cups chicken broth, preferably homemade
½ cup celery ribs, chopped
2 green garlic stalks, chopped 2 green onion stalks, chopped
1 ripe tomato, puréed
Kosher salt, to season
¼ teaspoon red pepper flakes
½ teaspoon Hungarian paprika
½ teaspoon ground black pepper
½ teaspoon mustard seeds
½ teaspoon sage
1 bay laurel

Directions:
Heat a stockpot over medium-high heat; once hot, fry the bacon until it is crisp or about 3 minutes. Add in the duck legs and cook until they are no longer pink.
Chop the meat, discarding any remaining skin and bones. Then, reserve the bacon and meat.
Pour in a splash of chicken broth to deglaze the pan.
Now, sauté the celery, green garlic and onions for 2 to 3 minutes, stirring periodically. Add the remaining ingredients to the pot, including the reserved bacon and meat.
Stir to combine and reduce the heat to medium-low. Let it cook, covered, until everything is thoroughly heated or about 1 hour. Serve in individual bowls and enjoy!

Nutrition:
calories: 364 | fat: 22.4g | protein: 33.2g | carbs: 5.1g | net carbs: 3.7g | fiber: 1.4g

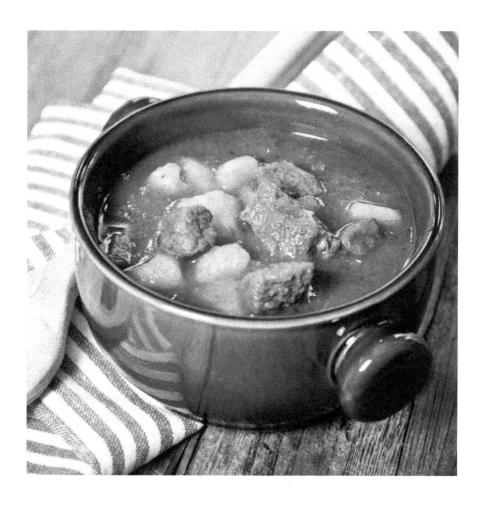

Chicken Rollatini

Preparation Time: 15 minutes
Cooking Time: 30 minutes
Servings: 4

Ingredients:
 4 (3-ounce) boneless skinless chicken breasts, pounded to about 1/3 inch thick
4 ounces ricotta cheese
4 slices prosciutto (4 ounces)
cup fresh spinach
1/2 cup almond flour
1/2 cup grated Parmesan cheese
eggs, beaten
1/4 cup good-quality olive oil

Directions:
Preheat the oven. Set the oven temperature to 400°F.
Prepare the chicken—Pat the chicken breasts dry with paper towels. Spread 1/4 of the ricotta in the middle of each breast. Place the prosciutto over the ricotta and 1/4 cup of the spinach on the prosciutto. Fold the long edges of the chicken breast over the filling, then roll the chicken breast up to enclose the filling. Place the rolls seam-side down on your work surface. Bread the chicken. On a plate, stir together the almond flour and Parmesan and set it next to the beaten eggs. Carefully dip a chicken roll in the egg, then roll it in the almond-flour mixture until it is completely covered. Set the rolls seam-side down on your work surface. Repeat with the other rolls. Brown the rolls. In a medium skillet over medium heat, warm the olive oil. Place the rolls seam-side down in the skillet and brown them on all sides, turning them carefully, about 10 minutes in total. Transfer the rolls, seam-side down, to a 9-by-9-inch baking dish—Bake the chicken rolls for 25 minutes, or until they're cooked through. Serve. Place one chicken roll on each of four plates and serve them immediately.

Nutrition:
Calories: 365; Fat: 17.1;gFiber: 9.4g; Carbohydrates:3.2 g; Protein: 1.

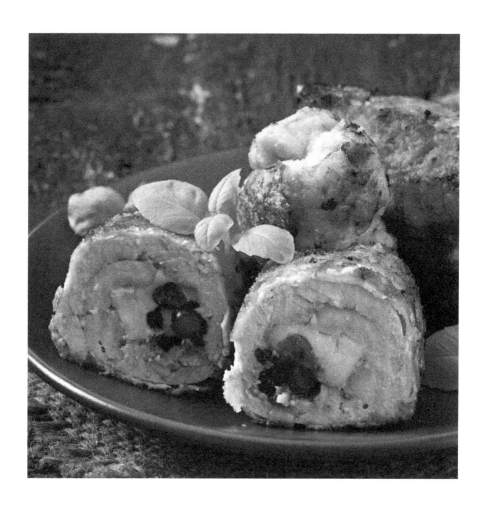

Indian Buttered Chicken

Preparation Time: 15 minutes
Cooking Time: 30 minutes
Servings: 4

Ingredients:
3 tablespoons unsalted butter
medium yellow onion, chopped
garlic cloves, minced
teaspoon fresh ginger, minced
11/2 pounds grass-fed chicken breasts, cut into 3/4-inch chunks
tomatoes, chopped finely1 tablespoon garam masala
1 teaspoon red chili powder
1 teaspoon ground cumin
Salt and ground black pepper, as required
cup heavy cream
tablespoons fresh cilantro, chopped

Directions:
In a wok, melt butter and sauté the onions for about 5–6 minutes.
Now, add in ginger and garlic and sauté for about 1 minute. Add the
tomatoes and cook for about 2–3 minutes, crushing with the back of
the spoon. Stir in the chicken spices, salt, and black pepper, and cook
for about 6–8 minutes or until the desired doneness of the chicken. Put
in the cream and cook for about 8–10 more minutes, stirring
occasionally. Garnish with fresh cilantro and serve hot.

Nutrition:
Calories: 456
Fat: 14.1g
Fiber: 10.5g
Carbohydrates:6.8 g
Protein: 12.8 g

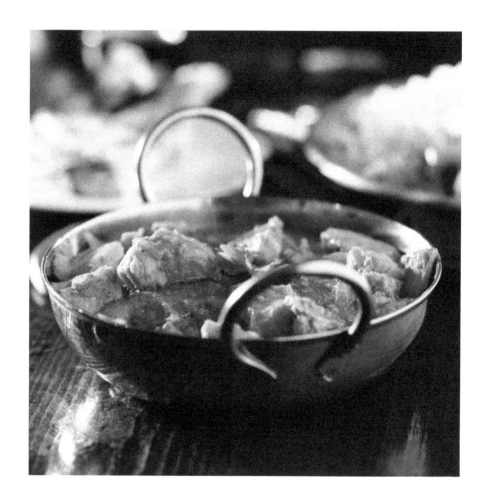

Chicken, Pepper, and Tomato Bake

Preparation time: 10 minutes
Cooking time: 25 minutes
Servings: 3

Ingredients:
tablespoon olive oil
¾ pound (340 g) chicken breast fillets, chopped into bite-sized chunks
garlic cloves, sliced
¼ teaspoon Korean chili pepper flakes
¼ teaspoon Himalayan salt
½ teaspoon poultry seasoning mix
bell pepper, deveined and chopped
ripe tomatoes, chopped
¼ cup heavy whipping cream
¼ cup sour cream

Directions:
Brush a casserole dish with olive oil. Add the chicken, garlic, Korean chili pepper flakes, salt, and poultry seasoning mix to the casserole dish.
Next, layer the pepper and tomatoes. Whisk the heavy whipping cream and sour cream in a mixing bowl.
Top everything with the cream mixture. Bake in the preheated oven at 390°F (199°C) for about 25 minutes or until thoroughly heated. Bon appétit!

Nutrition:
calories: 411
fat: 20.6g
protein: 50.0g
carbs: 6.2g
net carbs: 4.7g
fiber: 1.5g

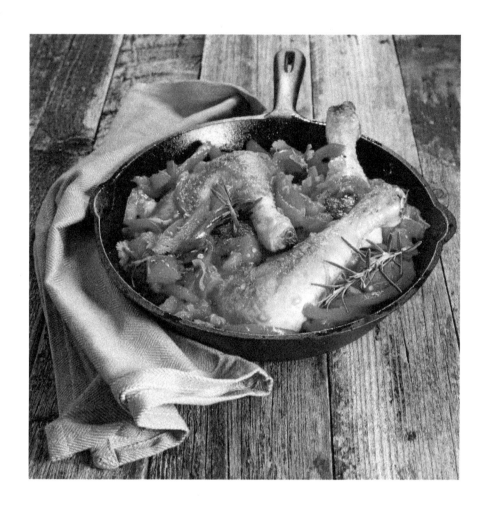

Roasted Whole Chicken with Black Olives

Preparation time: 10 minutes
Cooking time: 1 hour 15 minutes
Servings: 5

Ingredients:

2 pounds (907 g) whole chicken

1 teaspoon paprika

1 teaspoon lemon zest, slivered

Kosher salt and freshly ground black pepper, to taste

1 cup oil-cured black olives, pitted

4 cloves garlic

1 bunch fresh thyme, leaves picked

Directions:

Begin by preheating your oven to 360°F (182°C). Then, spritz the sides and bottom of a baking dish with nonstick cooking oil.

Sprinkle the chicken with paprika, lemon zest, salt, and black pepper. Bake for 60 minutes.

Scatter black olives, garlic, and thyme around the chicken and bake an additional 10 to 13 minutes; a meat thermometer should read 180°F (82°C). Bon appétit!

Nutrition:

calories: 236

fat: 7.4g

protein: 37.1g

carbs: 2.6g

net carbs: 1.6g

fiber: 1.0g

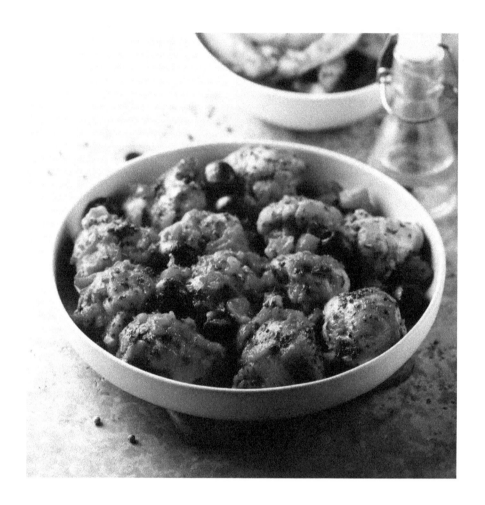

Pork

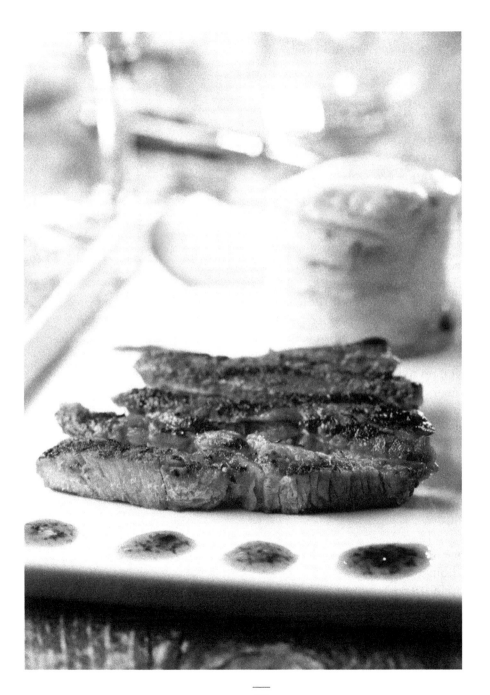

Sticky Pork Ribs

Preparation Time: 25 minutes
Cooking Time: 90 minutes
Servings: 8

Ingredients:
1/4 cups granulated erythritol
1 tablespoon garlic powder
1 tablespoon paprika
1/2 teaspoon red chili powder
4 pounds pork ribs, membrane removed
Salt and ground black pepper, as required
11/2 teaspoons liquid smoke 11/2 cups sugar-free BBQ sauce

Directions:
Preheat your oven to 300°F.
In a bowl, mix well erythritol, garlic powder, paprika, and chili powder. Season the ribs with pepper and salt. And then coat with the liquid smoke. Now, rub the ribs evenly with erythritol mixture. Arrange ribs onto the prepared baking sheet, meaty side down. Arrange two layers of foil on top of ribs and then roll and crimp edges tightly. Bake for about 2–21/2 hours or until the desired doneness. Now, set the oven to broiler. With a sharp knife, cut the ribs into serving-sized portions and evenly coat with the barbecue sauce. Arrange the ribs onto a broiler pan, bony side up. Broil for about 1–2 minutes per side. Remove from the oven and serve hot.

Nutrition:
Calories: 415
Fat: 18.1g
Fiber: 12.5g
Carbohydrates:3.1 g
Protein: 18.5g

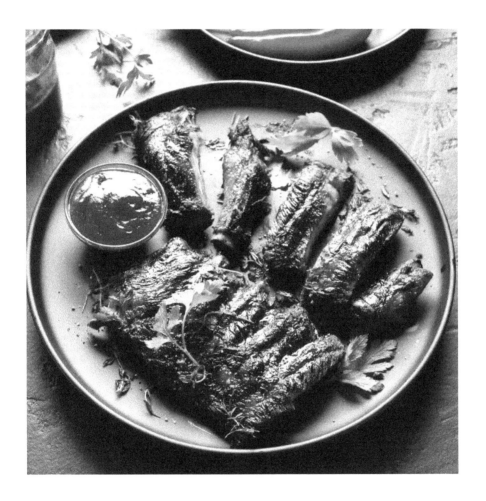

Herbed Grilled Lamb

Preparation Time: 15 minutes
Cooking Time: 20 minutes
Servings: 6

Ingredients:
 2 pounds of lamb
5 spoons of ghee butter
3 tablespoons of Keto mustard
2 minced garlic cloves
1 1/2 tablespoon of chopped basil
1/2 tablespoon of pepper
3 tablespoons of olive oil
1/2 teaspoon of salt

Directions:
Mix butter, mustard, and basil with a pinch of salt to taste. Then, set aside.
Mix garlic, salt, and pepper together. Then, add a teaspoon of oil.
Season the lamb generously with this mix.
Grill the lamb on medium heat until fully cooked.
Take butter mix and spread generously on chops and serve hot.

Nutrition:
Calories: 390
Fat: 19.5 g
Fiber: 5.9g
Carbohydrates: 3.2 g
Protein: 18.6 g

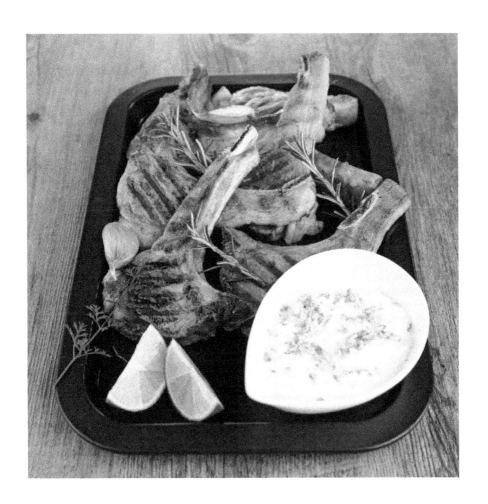

Pesto Pork Sausage Links

Preparation time: 10 minutes
Cooking time: 10 minutes
Servings: 8

Ingredients:
8 pork sausage links, sliced
1 pound (454 g) mixed cherry tomatoes, cut in half
4 cups baby spinach
1 tablespoon olive oil
pound (454 g) Monterrey Jack cheese, cubed
tablespoons lemon juice
1 cup basil pesto
Salt and black pepper, to taste

Direction:
Warm oil in a pan and cook sausage links for 4 minutes per side. In a salad bowl, combine spinach, cheese, salt, pesto, pepper, cherry tomatoes, and lemon juice, and toss to coat. Mix in the sausage.

Nutrition:
calories: 366
fat: 26.1g
protein: 17.9g
carbs: 8.0g
net carbs: 6.7g
fiber: 1.3g

BBQ Pork Ribs

Preparation time: 15 minutes
Cookimg time: 7 hours 5 minutes
Servings: 6

Ingredients:
3 racks pork ribs, silver lining removed
2 cups sugar-free BBQ sauce
2 tablespoons erythritol
2 teaspoons chili powder
2 teaspoons cumin powder
2 teaspoons onion powder
2 teaspoons smoked paprika
2 teaspoons garlic powder
Salt and black pepper to taste
1 teaspoon mustard powder
Preheat a smoker to 400°F (205°C) using mesquite wood to create flavor in the smoker.

Directions:
In a bowl, mix the erythritol, chili powder, cumin powder, black pepper, onion powder, smoked paprika, garlic powder, salt, and mustard powder. Rub the ribs and let marinate for 30 minutes.
Place on the grill grate, and cook at reduced heat of 225°F (107°C) for 4 hours. Flip the ribs after and continue cooking for 4 hours. Brush the ribs with BBQ sauce on both sides and sear them in increased heat for 3 minutes per side. Remove and let sit for 4 minutes before slicing. Serve with red cabbage coleslaw.

nutrition:
calories: 581
fat: 36.5g
protein: 44.6g
carbs: 1.8g
net carbs: 0g
fiber: 1.8g

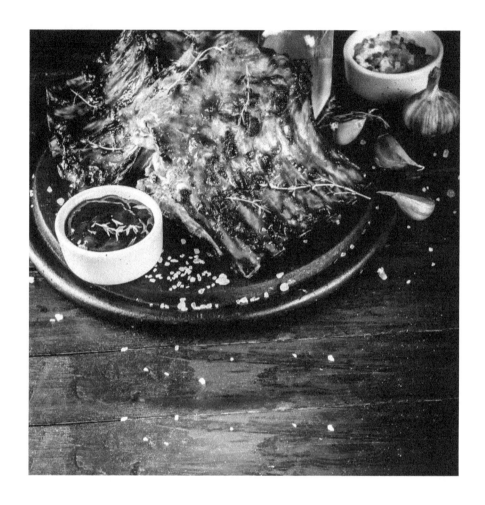

Pork and Mixed Vegetable Stir-Fry

Preparation time: 10 minutes
Cooking time: 20 minutes
ServIngs: 4

Ingredients:
1½ tablespoons butter
2 pounds (907 g) pork loin, cut into strips
Pink salt and chili pepper to taste
2 teaspoons ginger-garlic paste
¼ cup chicken broth
5 tablespoons peanut butter
2 cups mixed stir-fry vegetables

Directions:
Melt the butter in a wok and mix the pork with salt, chili pepper, and ginger-garlic paste. Pour the pork into the wok and cook for 6 minutes until no longer pink.
Mix the peanut butter with some broth until smooth, add to the pork and stir; cook for 2 minutes. Pour in the remaining broth, cook for 4 minutes, and add the mixed veggies. Simmer for 5 minutes. Adjust the taste with salt and black pepper, and spoon the stir-fry to a side of cilantro cauli rice.

Nutrition:
calories: 572
fat: 49.1g
protein: 22.6g
carbs:5.3 g
net carbs: 1.1g
fiber: 4.2g

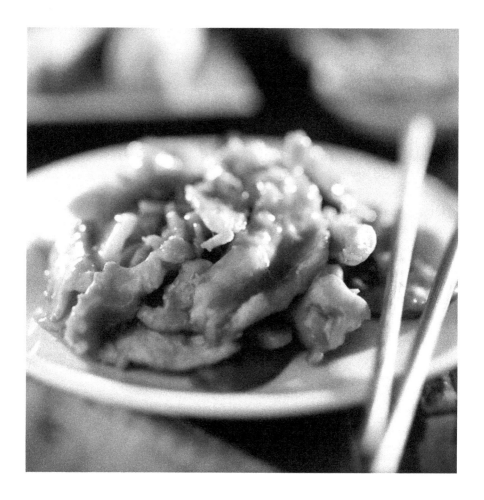

Beef and Lamb

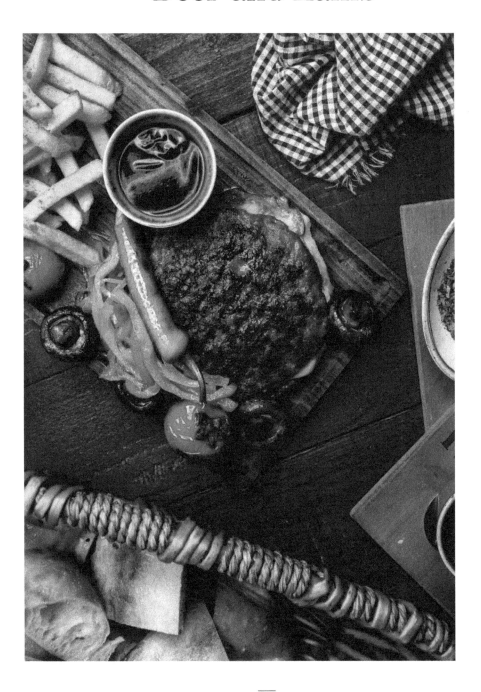

Bacon and Beef Stew

Preparation time: 15 minutes
Cooking time: 1 hour 10 minutes
Servings: 6

Ingredients:
8 ounces (227 g) bacon, chopped
4 pounds (1.8 kg) beef meat for stew, cubed
4 garlic cloves, minced
2 brown onions, chopped
2 tablespoons olive oil
4 tablespoons red vinegar
4 cups beef stock
2 tablespoons tomato purée
cinnamon sticks
lemon peel strips
½ cup fresh parsley, chopped
thyme sprigs
2 tablespoons butter
Salt and black pepper, to taste

Directions:
Set a saucepan over medium heat and warm oil, add in the garlic, bacon, and onion, and cook for 5 minutes. Stir in the beef, and cook until slightly brown. Pour in the vinegar, black pepper, butter, lemon peel strips, stock, salt, tomato purée, cinnamon sticks and thyme; stir for 3 minutes.
Cook for 1 hour while covered. Get rid of the thyme, lemon peel, and cinnamon sticks. Split into serving bowls and sprinkle with parsley to serve.

Nutrition:
calories: 591
fat: 36.1g
protein: 63.1g
carbs: 8.1g
net carbs: 5.6g
fiber: 2.5g

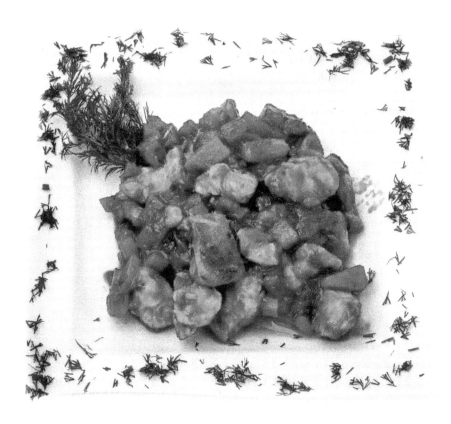

Pepperoni and Beef Pizza Meatloaf

Preparation time: 10 minutes
Cooking time: 60 minutes
Servings: 8

Ingredients:
2 pounds (907 g) ground beef (80/20)
⅓ cup superfine blanched almond flour
¼ cup grated Parmesan cheese
1 tablespoon dried parsley
1 tablespoon dried onion flakes
teaspoon kosher salt
½ teaspoon dried oregano leaves
½ teaspoon garlic powder
½ teaspoon ground black pepper
large eggs
cup marinara sauce, store-bought or homemade, plus more for serving if desired
cups shredded whole-milk Mozzarella cheese
4 ounces (113 g) thinly sliced pepperoni
Chopped fresh parsley, for garnish (optional)

Direction:
Preheat the oven to 375°F (190°C). Line a 9 by 5-inch loaf pan with foil, leaving 2 inches of foil folded over the outside edges of the pan. The extra foil will make it easier to lift the cooked meatloaf out of the pan. Place the ground beef, almond flour, Parmesan cheese, parsley, onion flakes, salt, oregano, garlic powder, pepper, and eggs in a large bowl and mix well by hand until the texture is uniform. Press the meatloaf mixture into the prepared loaf pan and flatten it out. Spoon the marinara evenly over the top and then sprinkle with the Mozzarella cheese. Layer the pepperoni slices on top. Bake, uncovered, for 1 hour, or until a meat thermometer inserted in the center reads 165°F (74°C).

Remove the meatloaf from the oven and let cool for at least 10 minutes in the pan to allow it to firm up before slicing. Carefully remove the meatloaf from the pan using the foil as handles. Place on a cutting board and remove the foil. You can then cut it into slices and serve on individual plates, or, to dress it up a bit, spread some warm marinara sauce on the bottom of a serving platter, then place the loaf on top of the sauce and garnish with fresh parsley, as shown.

Nutrition:
calories: 440
fat: 30.9g
protein: 32.8g
carbs: 3.4g
net carbs: 2.4g
fiber: 1.0g

Preparation time: 10 minutes
Cooking time: 35 minutes
Servings: 6

Ingredients:
1½ pounds (680 g) beef flank steak
Salt and black pepper to taste
1 cup crumbled Feta cheese
½ loose cup baby spinach
1 jalapeño pepper, chopped ¼ cup chopped basil leaves
Preheat oven to 400°F (205°C) and grease a baking sheet with cooking spray.

Directions:
Wrap the steak in plastic wrap, place on a flat surface, and gently run a rolling pin over to flatten. Take off the wraps. Sprinkle with half of the Feta cheese, top with spinach, jalapeño, basil leaves, and the remaining cheese. Roll the steak over on the stuffing and secure with toothpicks.
Place in the baking sheet and cook for 30 minutes, flipping once until nicely browned on the outside and the cheese melted within. Cool for 3 minutes, slice into pinwheels and serve with sautéed veggies.

Nutrition:
calories: 491
fat: 41.0g
protein: 28.0g
carbs: 2.1g
net carbs: 2.0g
fiber: 0.1g

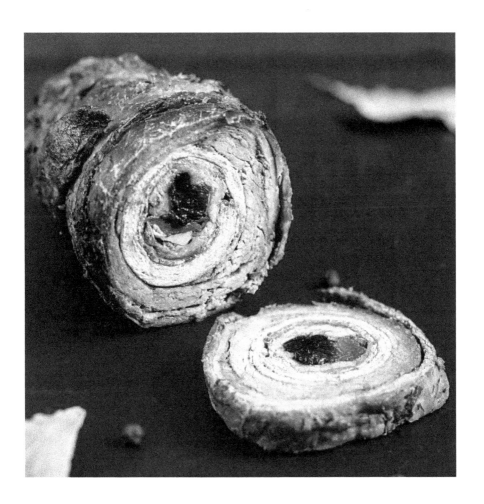

Lamb Curry

Preparation time: 15 minutes
Cooking time: 7 to 8 hours
Servings: 6

Ingredients:
3 tablespoons extra-virgin olive oil, divided
1½ pounds (680 g) lamb shoulder chops
Salt, for seasoning
Freshly ground black pepper, for seasoning
3 cups coconut milk
½ sweet onion, sliced
¼ cup curry powder
tablespoon grated fresh ginger
teaspoons minced garlic
carrot, diced
tablespoons chopped cilantro, for garnish

Directions:
Lightly grease the insert of the slow cooker with 1 tablespoon of the olive oil.
In a large skillet over medium-high heat, heat the remaining 2 tablespoons of the olive oil.
Season the lamb with salt and pepper. Add the lamb to the skillet and brown for 6 minutes, turning once. Transfer to the insert.
In a medium bowl, stir together the coconut milk, onion, curry, ginger, and garlic.
Add the mixture to the lamb along with the carrot.
Cover and cook on low for 7 to 8 hours.
Serve topped with the cilantro.

Nutrition:
calories: 491
fat: 41.2g
protein: 25.9g
carbs: 10.1g
net carbs: 5.2g
fiber: 4.9g

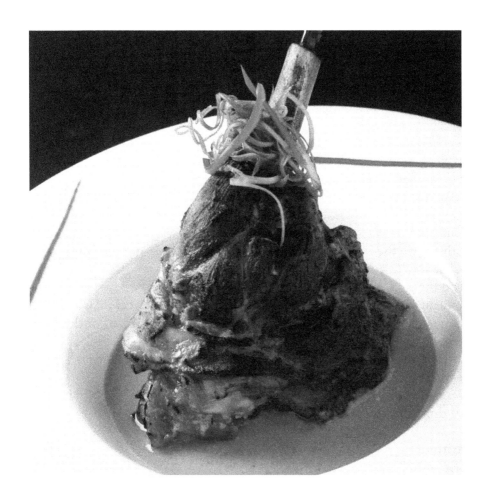

Lamb Chops with Fennel and Zucchini

Preparation time: 10 minutes
Cooking time: 6 hours
Servings: 4

Ingreedients:
¼ cup extra-virgin olive oil, divided
1 pound (454 g) boneless lamb chops, about ½-inch thick
Salt, for seasoning
Freshly ground black pepper, for seasoning
½ sweet onion, sliced
½ fennel bulb, cut into 2-inch chunks
zucchini, cut into 1-inch chunks
¼ cup chicken broth
tablespoons chopped fresh basil, for garnish

Directions:
Lightly grease the insert of the slow cooker with 1 tablespoon of the olive oil.
Season the lamb with salt and pepper.
In a medium bowl, toss together the onion, fennel, and zucchini with the remaining 3 tablespoons of the olive oil and then place half of the vegetables in the insert.
Place the lamb on top of the vegetables, cover with the remaining vegetables, and add the broth.
Cover and cook on low for 6 hours.
Serve topped with the basil.

Nutrition:
calories: 430
fat: 36.9g
protein: 20.9g
carbs: 5.0g
net carbs: 3.0g
fiber: 2.0g

Fish and Seafood

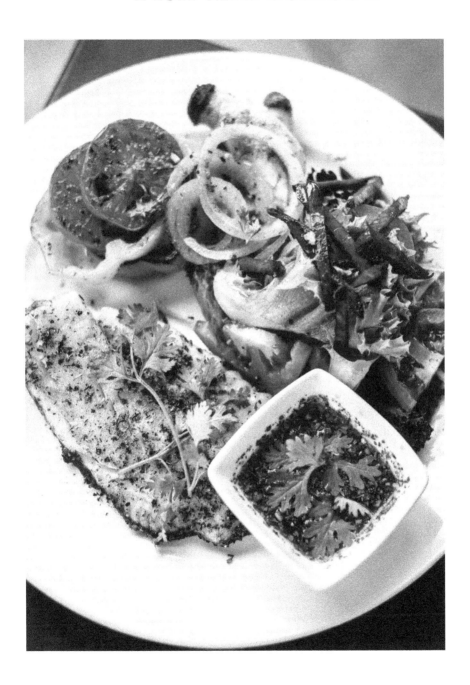

Asparagus and Trout Foil Packets

Preparation time: 15 minutes
Cooking time: 15 minutes
Servings: 4

Ingredients:
1 pound (454 g) asparagus spears
1 tablespoon garlic purée
1 pound (454 g) deboned trout, butterflied
Salt and black pepper to taste
3 tablespoons olive oil
2 sprigs rosemary
2 sprigs thyme
2 tablespoons butter
½ medium red onion, sliced
2 lemon slices
Preheat the oven to 400°F (205°C). Rub the trout with garlic purée, salt and black pepper.

Directions:
Prepare two aluminum foil squares. Place the fish on each square. Divide the asparagus and onion between the squares, top with a pinch of salt and pepper, a sprig of rosemary and thyme, and 1 tablespoon of butter. Also, lay the lemon slices on the fish. Wrap and close the fish packets securely, and place them on a baking sheet. Bake in the oven
for 15 minutes, and remove once ready.

Nutrition:
calories: 495
fat: 39.2g
protein: 26.9g
carbs: 7.5g
net carbs: 4.9g
fiber: 2.6g

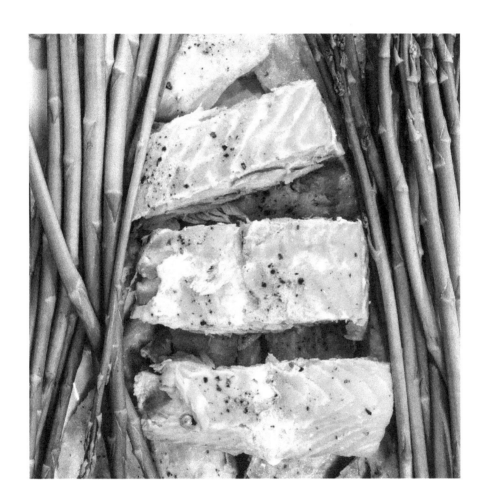

Shrimp Scampi

Preparation time: 5 minutes
Cooking time: 4 hours
Servings: 4

Ingredients:
1-pound shrimps, peeled
2 tablespoons lemon juice
2 tablespoons coconut oil
1 cup of water
1 teaspoon dried parsley
½ teaspoon white pepper

Directions
Put all ingredients in the slow cooker and gently mix.
Close the lid and cook the scampi on Low for 4 hours.

Nutrition
196 calories,
25.9g protein,
2.1g carbohydrates,
8.8g fat,
0.1g fiber,
239mg cholesterol,
280mg sodium,
207mg potassium

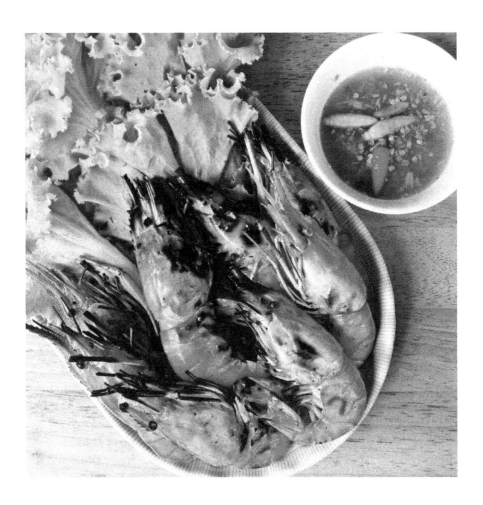

Tempura Zucchini with Cream Cheese Dip

Preparation Time: 15 minutes
Cooking Time: 15 minutes
Servings: 4

Ingredients:
Tempura zucchinis:
 1/2 cups (200 g) almond flour
tbsp. heavy cream
tsp. salt
tbsp. olive oil + extra for frying
1/4 cups (300 ml) water
1/2 tbsp. sugar-free maple syrup
large zucchinis, cut into 1-inch thick strips
Cream cheese dip:
8 oz cream cheese, room temperature
1/2 cup (113 g) sour cream
1 tsp. taco seasoning
1 scallion, chopped
1 green chili, deseeded and minced

Directions:
Tempura zucchinis:
In a bowl, mix the almond flour, heavy cream, salt, peanut oil, water, and maple syrup. Dredge the zucchini strips in the mixture until well-coated. Heat about four tablespoons of olive oil in a non-stick skillet. Working in batches, use tongs to remove the zucchinis (draining extra liquid) into the oil. Fry per side for 1 to 2 minutes and remove the zucchinis onto a paper towel-lined plate to drain grease. Enjoy the zucchinis.
Cream cheese dip:
In a bowl or container, the cream cheese, taco seasoning, sour cream, scallion, and green chili must be mixed, Serve the tempura zucchinis with the cream cheese dip.

Nutrition:
Calories: 316; Fat: 8.4g; Fiber: 9.3g; Carbohydrates:4.1 g; Protein: 5.1g

Shirataki Noodles with Grilled Tuna

Preparation time: 10 minutes
Cooking time: 25 minutes
Servings: 4

Ingredients:
1 (7-ounce / 198-g) pack shirataki noodles
3 cups water
1 red bell pepper, seeded and halved
4 tuna steaks
Salt and black pepper to taste
Olive oil for brushing
2 tablespoons pickled ginger
2 tablespoons chopped cilantro

Directions:
In a colander, rinse the shirataki noodles with running cold water.
Bring a pot of salted water to a boil; blanch the noodles for 2 minutes. Drain and transfer to a dry skillet over medium heat. Dry roast for a minute until opaque.
Grease a grill's grate with cooking spray and preheat on medium heat. Season the red bell pepper and tuna with salt and black pepper, brush with olive oil, and grill covered. Cook both for 3 minutes on each side. Transfer to a plate to cool. Dice bell pepper with a knife.
Assemble the noodles, tuna, and bell pepper in serving plate. Top with pickled ginger and garnish with cilantro. Serve with roasted sesame sauce.

Nutrition:
calories: 312
fat: 18.3g
protein: 22.1g
carbs: 2.5g
net carbs: 1.8g
fiber: 0.7g

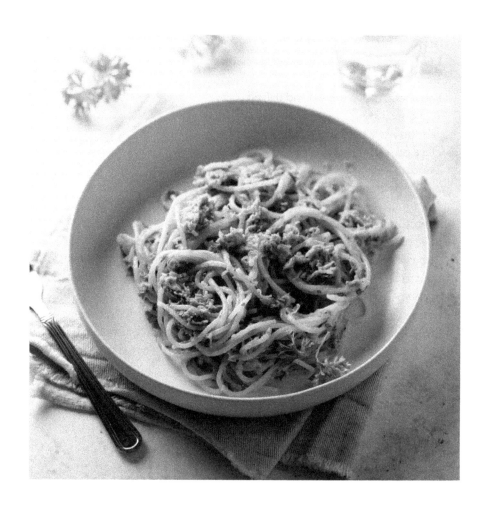

Salmon Fillets with Broccoli

Preparation time: 10 minutes
Cooking time: 30 minutes
Servings: 4

Ingredients:
4 salmon fillets
Salt and black pepper to taste
2 tablespoons mayonnaise
2 tablespoons fennel seeds, crushed
½ head broccoli, cut in florets
1 red bell pepper, sliced
tablespoon olive oil
lemon wedges

Directions:
Brush the salmon with mayonnaise and season with salt and black pepper. Coat with fennel seeds, place in a lined baking dish and bake for 15 minutes at 370°F (188°C). Steam the broccoli and carrot for 3-4 minutes, or until tender, in a pot over medium heat.
Heat the olive oil in a saucepan and sauté the red bell pepper for 5 minutes. Stir in the broccoli and turn off the heat. Let the pan sit on the warm burner for 2-3 minutes. Serve with baked salmon garnished with lemon wedges.

Nutritio:
calories: 564
fat: 36.8g
protein: 53.9g
carbs: 8.3g
net carbs: 5.9g
fiber: 2.4g

Salads

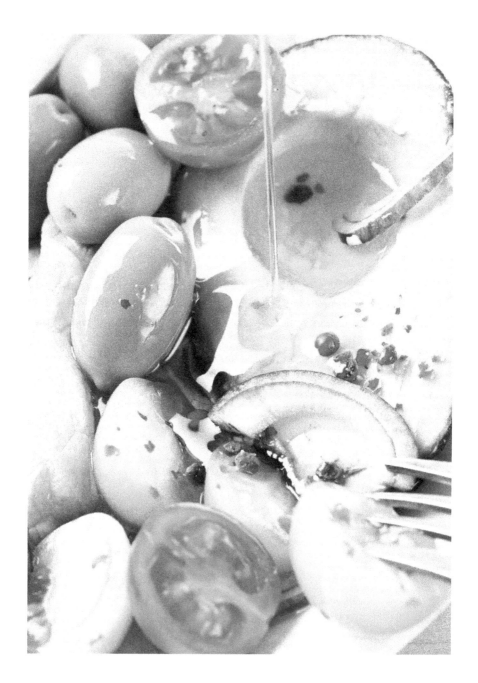

Kale and Smoked Salmon Salad

Preparation time: 15 minutes
Cooking time: 0 minutes
Servings: 4

Ingredients:
¼ cup extra virgin olive oil
1 tablespoon lemon juice
½ teaspoon garlic powder
½ teaspoon sea salt
¼ teaspoon black pepper
6 ounces (170 g) chopped and deribbed kale (from 8 to 10 ounces / 227 to 283 g untrimmed)
¼ cup salted roasted sunflower seeds
8 ounces (227 g) smoked salmon, cut into pieces

Directions:
In a large bowl, whisk together the olive oil, lemon juice, garlic powder, sea salt, and black pepper.
Add the chopped kale. Use your hands to massage the kale with the dressing mixture. Grab a bunch, squeeze with the dressing, release, and repeat. Do this for a couple of minutes, until the kale starts to soften.
Add the sunflower seeds and smoked salmon. Toss together.

Nutrition:
calories: 258
fat: 20.0g
protein: 14.0g
carbs: 6.0g
net carbs: 6.0g
fiber: 0g

Feta Cucumber Salad

Preparation time: 10 minutes
Cooking time: 0 minutes
Servings: 5

Ingredients:
2 medium-large cucumbers
½ cup thinly sliced red onions
4 ounces (113 g) Feta cheese, crumbled
Salt and pepper to taste
Dressing:
¼ cup extra-virgin olive oil
1 tablespoon red wine vinegar
1 tablespoon Swerve confectioners'-style sweetener
½ teaspoon dried ground oregano

Directions:
Peel the cucumbers as desired and cut in half lengthwise, then slice.
In a medium-sized bowl, toss the cucumbers with the onions. Add the Feta and gently toss to combine.
Make the dressing: Place all the ingredients in a small bowl and whisk to combine.
Serve right away or place in the refrigerator to chill before serving. To serve, gently toss the salad with the dressing and season to taste with salt and pepper.

Nutrition:
calories: 172
fat: 15.2g
protein: 4.5g
carbs: 6.5g
net carbs: 3.7g
fiber: 2.8g

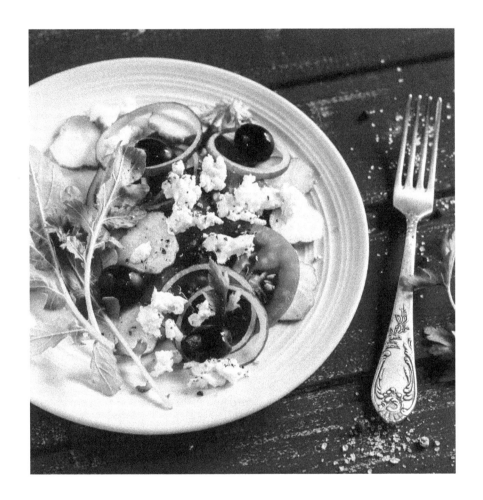

Mediterranean Tomato and Zucchini Salad

Preparation time: 15 minutes
Cooking time: 10 minutes
Servings: 4

Ingredients:
½ pound (227 g) Roma tomatoes, sliced
½ pound (227 g) zucchini, sliced
1 Lebanese cucumber, sliced
1 cup arugula
½ teaspoon oregano
½ teaspoon basil
½ teaspoon rosemary
½ teaspoon ground black pepper
Sea salt, to season
4 tablespoons extra-virgin olive oil
2 tablespoons fresh lemon juice
½ cup Kalamata olives, pitted and sliced
4 ounces (113 g) Feta cheese, cubed

Directions:
Arrange the Roma tomatoes and zucchini slices on a roasting pan;
spritz cooking oil over your vegetables.
Bake in the preheated oven at 350°F (180°C) for 6 to 7 minutes. Let
them cool slightly, then, transfer to a salad bowl.
Add in the cucumber, arugula, herbs, and spices. Drizzle olive oil and
lemon juice over your veggies; toss to combine well.
Top with Kalamata olives and Feta cheese. Serve at room temperature
and enjoy!

Nutrition:
calories: 242
fat: 22.1g
protein: 6.4g
carbs: 6.9g
net carbs: 5.1g
fiber: 1.8g

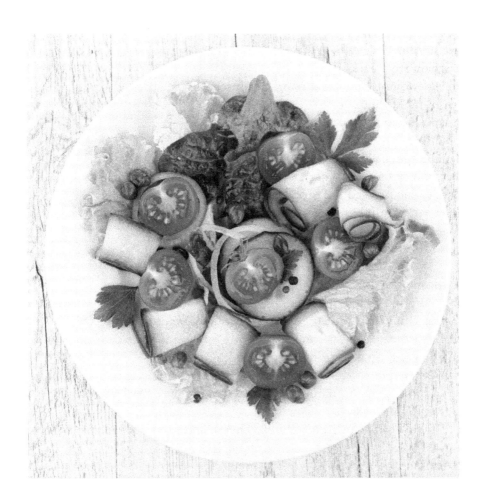

Asparagus and Mozzarella Caprese Salad

Preparation time: 15 minutes
Cooking time: 0 minutes
Servings: 2

Ingredients:
1 teaspoon fresh lime juice
1 tablespoon hot Hungarian paprika infused oil
½ teaspoon kosher salt
¼ teaspoon red pepper flakes
½ pound (227 g) asparagus spears, trimmed
cup grape tomatoes, halved
tablespoon red wine vinegar
1 garlic clove, pressed 1-2 drops liquid stevia
1 tablespoon fresh basil
1 tablespoon fresh chives
½ cup Mozzarella, grated

Directions:
Heat your grill to the hottest setting. Toss your asparagus with the lime juice, hot Hungarian paprika infused oil, salt, and red pepper flakes. Place the asparagus spears on the hot grill. Grill until one side chars; then, grill your asparagus on the other side.
Cut the asparagus spears into bite-sized pieces and transfer to a salad bowl. Add the grape tomatoes, red wine, garlic, stevia, basil, and chives; toss to combine well.
4. Top with freshly grated Mozzarella cheese and serve immediately.

Nutrition:
calories: 190
fat: 13.2g
protein: 9.6g
carbs: 7.5g
net carbs: 4.2g
fiber: 3.3g

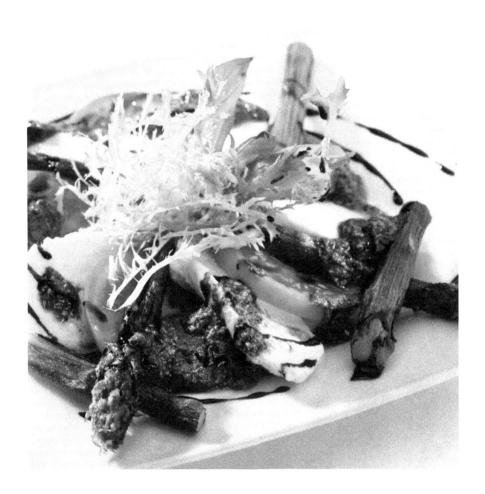

Soups

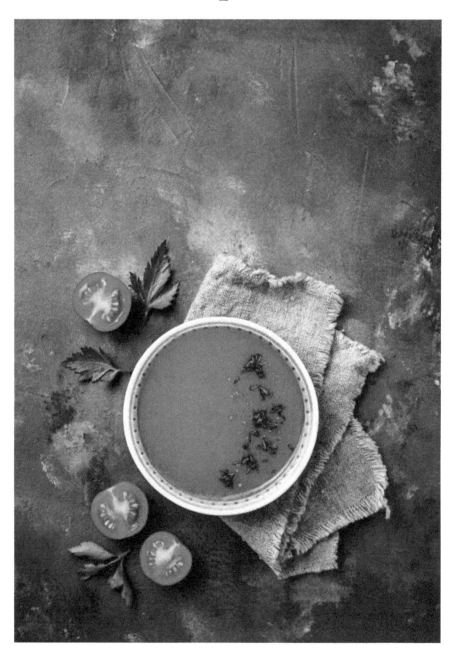

Chicken Lemon Soup

Preparation time: 10 minutes
Cooking time: 4 hours
Servings: 6

Ingredients:
6 cups chicken broth
3 boneless, skinless chicken breasts
Juice from 1 lemon
yellow onion, chopped
cloves garlic, chopped
1 teaspoon cayenne pepper
1 teaspoon dried thyme
1 handful of fresh parsley, minced
Salt and black pepper, to taste

Directions:
Add all the ingredients minus the salt, black pepper and parsley to the base of a slow cooker minus the parsley and cook on high for 4 hours.
Add the parsley and season with salt and black pepper.
Shred the chicken and serve.

Nutrition:
calories: 110
fat: 3.0g
protein: 15.9g
carbs: 4.1g
net carbs: 2.9g
fiber: 1.2g

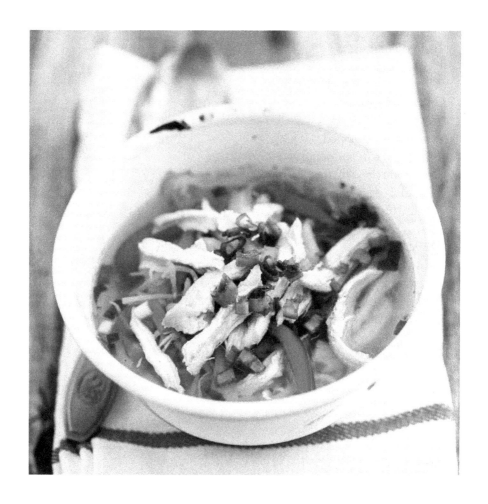

Roasted Tomato and Cheddar Soup

Preparation Time: 10 minutes
Cooking Time: 15-20 minutes
Servings: 4

Ingredients:
2 tbsp. butter
2 medium yellow onions, sliced
garlic cloves, minced
thyme sprigs
8 basil leaves + extra for garnish
8 tomatoes
1/2 tsp. red chili flakes
2 cups vegetable broth
Salt and black pepper to taste
1 cup grated cheddar cheese (white and sharp)

Directions:
Melt the butter in a pot and sauté the onions and garlic for 3 minutes or until softened. Stir in the thyme, basil, tomatoes, red chili flakes, and vegetable broth.
Season with salt and black pepper. Boil it then simmer for 10 minutes or until the tomatoes soften. Puree all ingredients until smooth. Season. Garnish with the cheddar cheese and basil. Serve warm.

Nutrition:
Calories: 341
Fat: 12.9g
Fiber: 9.6g
Carbohydrates:4.8 g
Protein: 4.1g

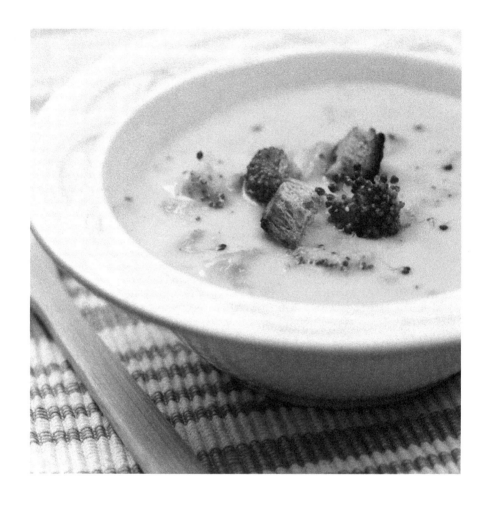

Nutmeg Pumpkin Soup

Preparation Time: 15 minutes
Cooking Time: 20 minutes
Servings: 4

Ingredients:
1 tablespoon of butter
1 onion (diced)
1 16-ounce can of pumpkin puree
1 1/3 cups of vegetable broth
1/2 tablespoon of nutmeg
1/2 tablespoon of sugar
Salt (to taste)
Pepper (to taste)
3 cups of soymilk or any milk as a substitute

Directions:
Using a large saucepan, add onion to margarine and cook it between 3 and 5 minutes until the onion is clear
Add pumpkin puree, vegetable broth, sugar, pepper, and other ingredients and stir to combine.
Cook in medium heat for between 10 and fifteen minutes
Before serving the soup, taste and add more spices, pepper, and salt if necessary Serve soup and enjoy it!

Nutrition:
Calories: 165
Fat: 4.9g
Fiber: 11.9g
Carbohydrates:3.5 g
Protein: 4.2g

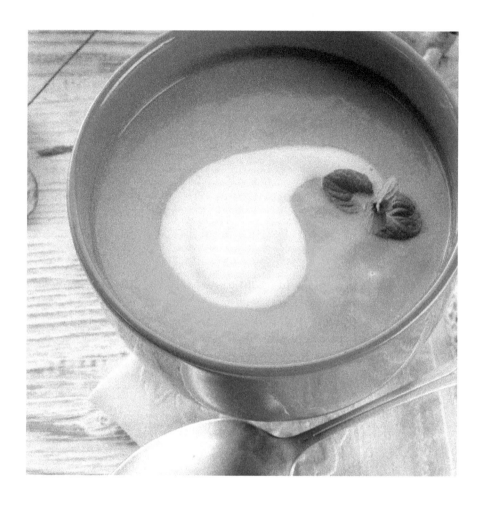

Broccoli Cheddar Soup

Preparation Time: 15 minutes
Cooking Time: 15 minutes
Servings: 2

Ingredients:
1/4 medium onion, chopped
2 tablespoons butter
1 garlic clove, minced
1 cup chicken broth
3/4 teaspoon pink Himalayan sea salt
1/2 teaspoon freshly ground black pepper
1/4 teaspoon dry mustard powder
8 ounces fresh broccoli florets, cooked and finely chopped
1 cup heavy (whipping) cream 1 cup shredded cheddar cheese

Directions:
In a medium pot, combine the onion, butter, and garlic over medium heat. Cook for 7 to 10 minutes until the onion is tender.
Add the broth, salt, pepper, and mustard, and bring the mixture to a boil.
Reduce the heat and add the broccoli and cream.
Slowly add the cheese, stirring. Serve.

Nutrition:
Calories: 317
Fat: 11.9g
Fiber: 9.5g
Carbohydrates:4.3 g
Protein: 8.5g

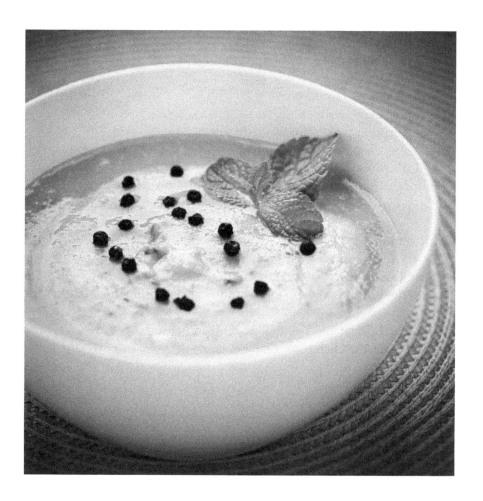

Shrimp Jalapeño Soup

Preparation time: 10 minutes
Cooking time: 35 minutes
Servings: 6

Ingredients:
4 cups chicken broth
Juice from 1 lime
1 pound (454 g) peeled, deveined shrimp
1 yellow onion, chopped
1 shallot, chopped
3 cloves garlic, chopped
1 jalapeño pepper, seeded and sliced
Salt and black pepper, to taste
1 tablespoon coconut oil for cooking

Directions:
Add the coconut oil to a large stockpot over medium heat.
Add the shrimp, onion, shallot and garlic and cook until the shrimp are cooked through and pink.
Add the remaining ingredients minus the salt and black pepper, and bring to a boil.
Reduce the heat to a simmer and cook for 30 minutes.
Season with salt and black pepper and serve.

Nutrition:
calories: 154
fat: 4.9g
protein: 21.2g
carbs: 5.9g
net carbs: 4.8g
fiber: 1.1g

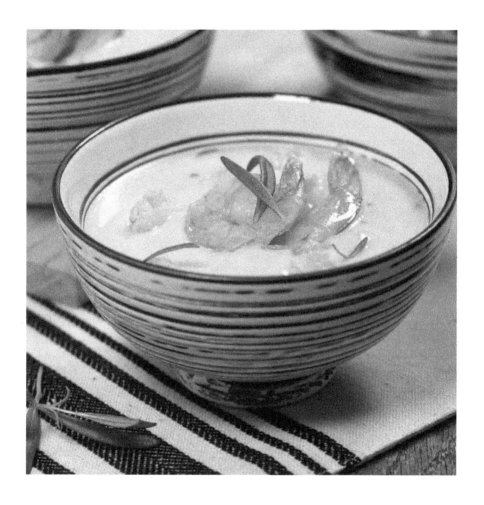

Snacks and Appetizers

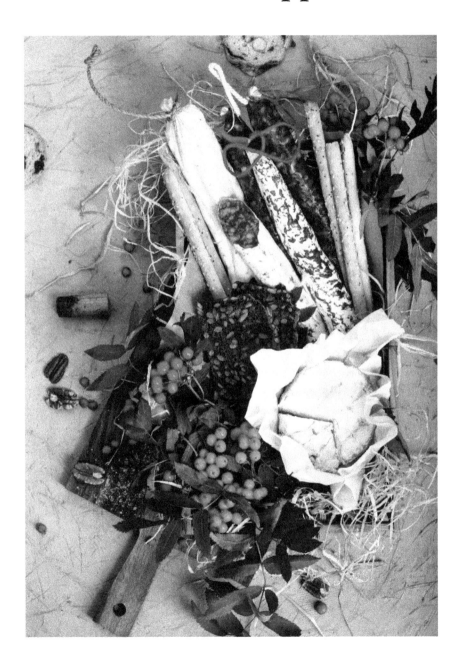

BLT Cups

Preparation time: 10 minutes
Cooking time: 10 minutes
Servings: 10

Ingredients:
5 ounces (142 g) bacon, chopped
5 tablespoons Parmigiano-Reggiano cheese, grated
teaspoon adobo sauce
tablespoons mayonnaise
Sea salt and ground black pepper, to taste
2 tablespoons green onions, minced
10 pieces lettuce
10 tomatoes cherry tomatoes, discard the insides

Direcctions:
Preheat a frying pan over moderate heat. Cook the bacon in the frying pan until crisp, about 7 minutes; reserve.
In a mixing bowl, thoroughly combine the cheese, adobo sauce, mayo, salt, black pepper, and green onions. Divide the mayo mixture between the cherry tomatoes.
Divide the cooked bacon between the cherry tomatoes. Top with the lettuce and serve immediately. Bon appétit!

Nutrition:
calories: 93
fat: 8.2g
protein: 2.6g
carbs: 1.5g
net carbs: 1.1g
fiber: 0.4g

Deviled Eggs

Preparation time: 10 minutes
Cooking time: 20 minutes
Servings: 6

Ingredients:
6 eggs
1 tablespoon green tabasco
⅓ cup sugar-free mayonnaise

Directions:
Place the eggs in a saucepan, and cover with salted water. Bring to a boil over medium heat. Boil for 8 minutes. Place the eggs in an ice bath and let cool for 10 minutes. Peel and slice them in. Whisk together the tabasco, mayonnaise, and salt in a small bowl. Spoon this mixture on top of every egg.

Nutrition:
calories: 180
fat: 17.0g
protein: 6.0g
carbs: 5.0g
net carbs: 5.0g
fiber: 0g

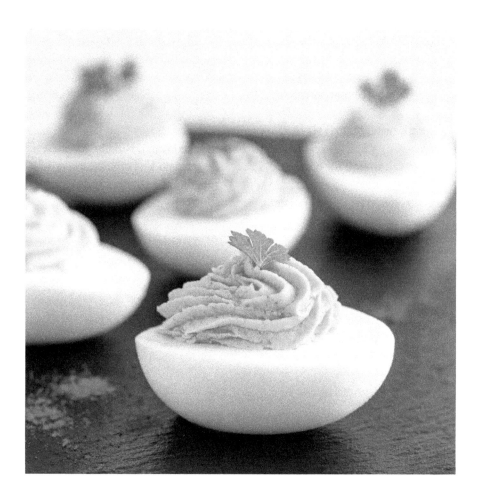

Strawberry Fat Bombs

Preparation Time: 30 minutes
Cooking Time: 0 minutes
Servings: 6

Ingredients:
100 g strawberries
100 g cream cheese
50 g butter
2 tbsp. erythritol powder 1/2 teaspoon vanilla extract

Directions:
Put the cream cheese and butter (cut into small pieces) in a mixing bowl.
Let rest for 30 to 60 minutes at room temperature.
In the meantime, wash the strawberries and remove the green parts.
Pour into a bowl and process into a puree with a serving of oil or a mixer.
Add erythritol powder and vanilla extract and mix well.
Mix the strawberries with the other ingredients and make sure that they have reached room temperature.
Put the cream cheese and butter into a container.
Mix with a hand mixer or a food processor to a homogeneous mass.
Pour the mixture into small silicone muffin molds. Freeze.

Nutrition:
Calories: 95
Fat: 9.1g
Fiber: 4.1g
Carbohydrates:0.9 g

Jalapeño and Zucchini Frittata Cups

Preparation time: 15 minutes
Cooking time: 30 minutes
Servings: 4

Ingredients:
2 tablespoons olive oil
2 green onions, chopped
1 garlic clove, minced
½ jalapeño pepper, chopped
½ carrot, chopped
zucchini, shredded
tablespoons Mozzarella cheese, shredded
8 eggs, whisked
Salt and black pepper, to taste
½ teaspoon dried oregano

Directions:
Sauté green onions and garlic in warm olive oil over medium heat for 3 minutes. Stir in carrot, zucchini, and jalapeño pepper, and cook for 4 more minutes. Remove the mixture to a lightly greased baking pan with a nonstick cooking spray. Top with Mozzarella cheese.
Cover with the whisked eggs; season with oregano, black pepper, and salt. Bake in the oven for about 20 minutes at 360°F (182°C).

Nutrition:
calories: 336
fat: 27.9g
protein: 14.1g
carbs: 5.3g
net carbs: 4.8g
fiber: 0.5g

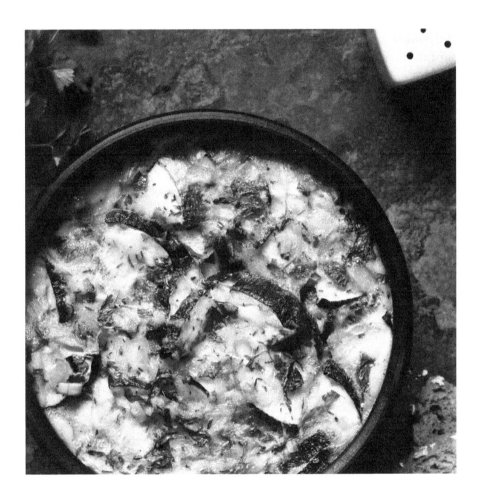

Thai Tofu Mix

Preparation time: 10 minutes
Cooking time: 10 hours
Servings: 2

Ingredients:
pound firm tofu, pressed and cut into rectangles
½ tablespoons sesame oil
tablespoon soy sauce
¼ cup veggie stock
½ cup pineapple juice
tablespoons rice vinegar
1 tablespoon sugar
½ tablespoon ginger, grated
1 garlic clove, minced
3 pineapple rings

Directions:
In your slow cooker, mix tofu with sesame oil, soy sauce, stock, pineapple juice, vinegar, sugar, ginger, garlic and pineapple rings, stir, cover and cook on Low for 10 hours.
Divide into bowls and serve as an appetizer.
Enjoy!

Nutrition
Calories 201,
Fat 5,
Fiber 7,
Carbs 15, Protein 4

Dessert

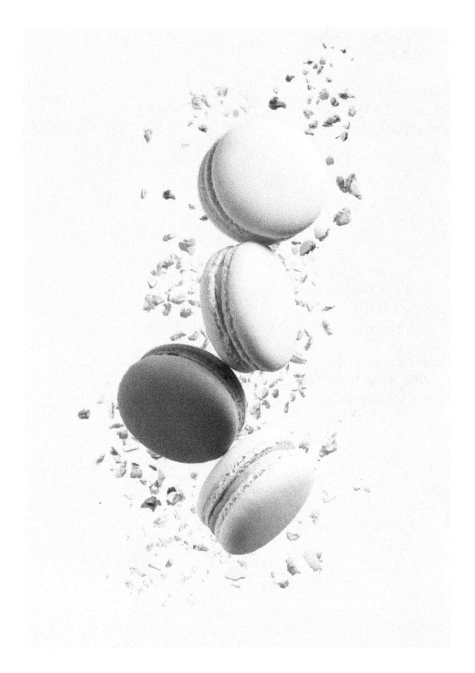

Green Tea and Macadamia Brownies

Preparation Time: 10 minutes
Cooking Time: 20 minutes
Servings: 4

Ingredients:
4 tablespoons Swerve confectioners style sweetener
1/4 cup unsalted butter, melted
Salt, to taste
1 egg
1 tablespoon tea matcha powder
1/4 cup coconut flour
1/2 teaspoon baking powder 1/2 cup chopped macadamia nuts

Directions:
Let the oven heat up to 350F.
Combine the sweetener, melted butter, and salt in a bowl. Stir to mix well. Separate the egg into the bowl, whisk to combine well. Fold in the matcha powder, coconut flour, and baking powder, then add the macadamia nuts. Stir to combine. Pour the mixture on a baking sheet Level the mixture with a spoon to make sure it coats the bottom of the sheet evenly. Bake for 18 minutes or until a sharp knife inserted in the center of the brownies comes out clean. Remove the brownies from the oven and slice to serve.

Nutrition:
Calories: 241
Fat: 15.9g
Fiber: 6.0g
Carbohydrates:12.1 g Protein: 9.6g

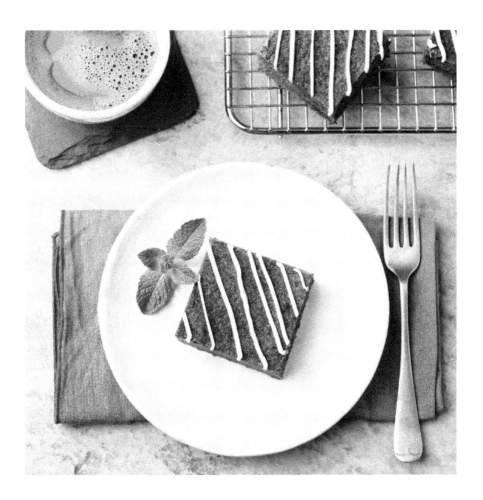

Tapioca and Chia Pudding

Preparation time: 10 minutes
Cooking time: 3 hours
Servings: 2

Ingredients:
cup almond milk
¼ cup tapioca pearls
tablespoons chia seeds
eggs, whisked
½ teaspoon vanilla extract
tablespoons sugar
½ tablespoon lemon zest, grated

Directions:
In your slow cooker, mix the tapioca pearls with the milk, eggs and the other ingredients, whisk, put the lid on and cook on Low for 3 hours.
Divide the pudding into bowls and serve cold.

Nutrition
Calories 180,
Fat 3,
Fiber 4,
Carbs 12, Protein 4

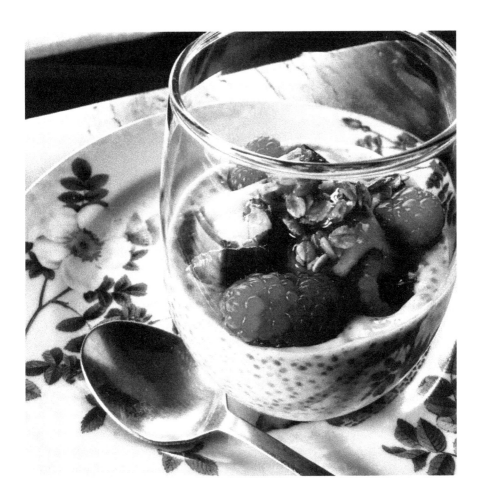

Rhubarb Bars

Preparation time: 10 minutes
Cooking time: 15 minutes
Servings: 4

Ingredients:
5 oz rhubarb, chopped
2 tablespoons liquid stevia
1 teaspoon swerve
1 teaspoon vanilla extract
tablespoons butter
4 tablespoons coconut flour
¼ teaspoon ground cinnamon

Directions:
Combine the liquid stevia, swerve, vanilla extract, butter, coconut flour, and ground cinnamon.
Knead into a smooth dough.
Place the dough in the slow cooker and flatten it into the shape of a pie crust.
Sprinkle with the chopped rhubarb and press gently.
Close the lid and cook the dessert for 3 hours.
Cool and cut into the bars.
Enjoy!

Nutrition:
calories 42,
fat 0.8,
fiber 3.7,
carbs 7.4,
protein 1.3

Snowball Cookies

Preparation time: 20 minutes
Cooking time: 2.5 hours
Servings: 6

Ingredients:
2 tablespoons coconut flakes, unsweetened
1 egg, beaten
4 tablespoons flour
2 tablespoons butter
1 tablespoon Erythritol
1 tablespoon water

Directions:
Mix the egg, flour, butter, Erythritol, and water.
Knead into a smooth dough.
Make small balls from the dough and coat them in the coconut flakes.
Place the cookies in the slow cooker and cook for 2.5 hours on High.
Chill the cookies and serve!

Nutrition:
calories 69,
fat 5.2,
fiber 0.3,
carbs 6.8,
protein 1.6

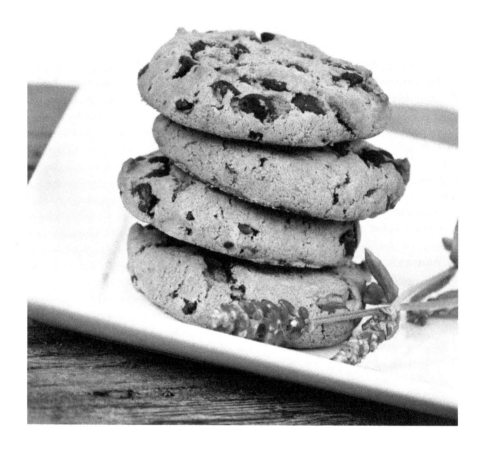

Avocado Bars

Preparation time: 20 minutes
Cooking time: 20 minutes
Servings: 6

Ingredients:
avocado, pitted
¾ cup coconut flour
1 teaspoon vanilla extract
tablespoons butter
tablespoons liquid stevia
tablespoons almond flour½ teaspoon baking powder

Directions:
Peel the avocado and mash it.
Combine the mashed avocado and coconut flour.
Add vanilla extract and butter.
After this, add liquid stevia, baking powder and almond flour.
Stir the mix until smooth and transfer in the slow cooker.
Flatten it gently and cook for 3 hours on High.
Cut the cooked dessert into bars and serve!

Nutrition:
calories 174,
fat 15.1,
fiber 5.8,
carbs 6,
protein 1.9

Keto Soufflé

Preparating time: 25 minutes
Cooking time: 2.5 hours
Servings: 5

Ingredients:
1 tablespoon butter
¼ cup Erythritol
1 oz dark chocolate
4 egg yolks
2 egg whites
5 teaspoon whipped cream

Directions:
Whisk the butter with Erythritol.
Add the egg yolks and stir until well blended.
Whisk the eggs to stiff peaks.
Melt the chocolate and combine it with the egg yolk mixture.
Add the egg whites and whipped cream.
Stir gently to get a smooth batter.
Place the mixture in ramekins and put the ramekins in the slow cooker.
Cook the soufflé for 2.5 hours on Low.
Serve it immediately!

Nutrition:
calories 115,
fat 9.2,
fiber 0.2,
carbs 16.1,
protein 4.2

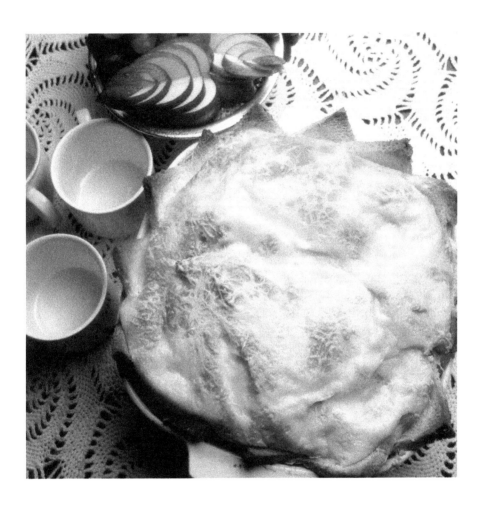

Walnut Muffins

Preparating time: 20 minutes
Cooking time: 3 hours
Servings: 8

Ingredients:
2 oz walnuts, chopped
5 tablespoons butter 1 cup coconut flour
1 teaspoon vanilla extract
egg
tablespoons liquid stevia
tablespoons almond milk, unsweetened
1 teaspoon baking powder

Directions:
Mix the butter, flour, vanilla extract, liquid stevia, almond milk, and baking powder.
Beat the egg into the mixture and whisk it well until smooth.
Add the chopped walnuts and stir well.
Place the dough in the muffin molds and transfer into the slow cooker.
Cook the muffins for 3 hours on High.
Cool the cooked muffins and enjoy!

Nutrition:
calories 190,
fat 14.8,
fiber 6.6,
carbs 11.4,
protein 4.6

Drinks

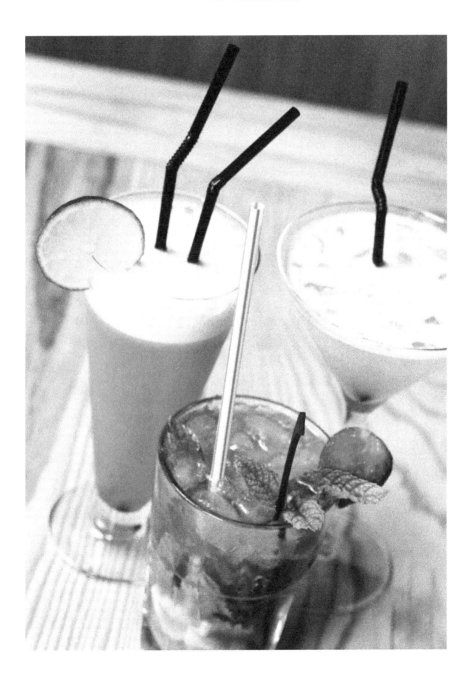

Kiwi Coconut Smoothie

Preparation Time: 5 minutes
Cooking Time: 0 minutes
Servings: 2

Ingredients:
2 kiwis, pulp scooped
1 tbsp. xylitol
4 ice cubes
2 cups unsweetened coconut milk
1 cup of coconut yogurt
Mint leaves to garnish

Directions:
Process the kiwis, xylitol, coconut milk, yogurt, and ice cubes in a blender, until smooth, for about 3 minutes.
Transfer to serving glasses, garnish with mint leaves, and serve.

Nutrition:
Calories: 298
Fat: 1.2g
Fiber: 12.1g
Carbohydrates:1.2 g
Protein: 3.2g

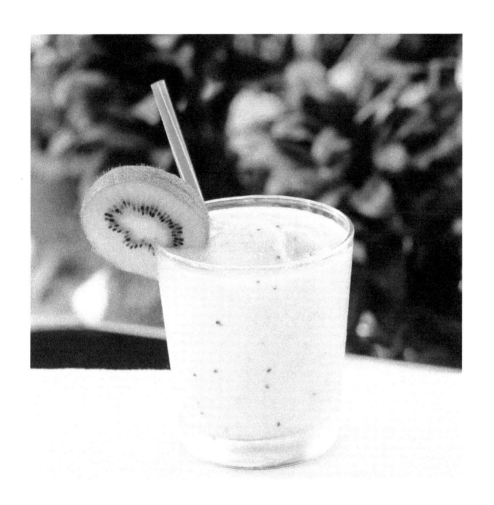

Lemony Caper Dressing

Preparation time: 5 minutes
Cooking time: 0 minutes
Makes: ¾ cup

Ingredients:
½ cup sugar-free mayonnaise
2 tablespoons extra-virgin olive oil
1 tablespoon capers, drained
1 tablespoon lemon juice
1 tablespoon white vinegar
1 teaspoon grated lemon zest
½ teaspoon dried dill weed

Directions:
Place all of the ingredients in a small blender and blend for 30 seconds, until creamy and nearly entirely smooth. Store in an airtight container in the refrigerator for up to 1 week.

Per Serving
calories: 106
fat: 13.0g
protein: 0g
carbs: 0g
net carbs: 0g
fiber: 0g

Dill Feta Dressing

Preparation time: 5 minutes
Cooking time: 0 minutes
Makes: 1 cup

Ingredients:
¼ cup sugar-free mayonnaise
⅓ cup crumbled Feta cheese
2 tablespoons full-fat sour cream
2 tablespoons heavy whipping cream
1 tablespoon chopped fresh dill
1 tablespoon white vinegar
⅛ teaspoon ground black pepper
⅛ teaspoon onion powder

Directions:
Place all of the ingredients in a small blender and blend for 30 seconds, until creamy and nearly entirely smooth. Store in an airtight container in the refrigerator for up to 1 week.

Nutrition:
calories: 75
fat: 8.1g
protein: 1.2g
carbs: 0.3g
net carbs: 0.3g
fiber: 0g

Creamy Cinnamon Smoothie

Preparation Time: 15 minutes
Cooking Time: 0 minutes
Servings: 2

Ingredients:
2 cups of coconut milk
1 scoop vanilla protein powder
5 drops liquid stevia
1 teaspoon ground cinnamon
1/2 teaspoon alcohol-free vanilla extract

Directions:
Put the coconut milk, protein powder, stevia, cinnamon, and vanilla in a blender and blend until smooth.
Pour into two glasses and serve immediately.

Nutrition:
Calories: 212
Fat: 3.1g
Fiber: 5.2g
Carbohydrates:3.7 g
Protein: 4.1g

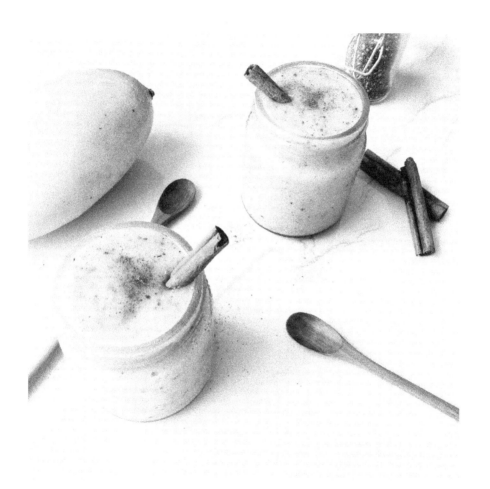

Creamy Vanilla Cappuccino

Preparation Time: 5 minutes
Cooking Time: 0 minutes
Servings: 2

Ingredients:
2 cups unsweetened vanilla almond milk, chilled
1 tsp. swerve sugar
1/2 tbsp. powdered coffee
1 cup cottage cheese, cold
1/2 tsp. vanilla bean paste
1/4 tsp. xanthan gum
Unsweetened chocolate shavings to garnish

Directions:
In a blender, combine the almond milk, swerve sugar, cottage cheese, coffee, vanilla bean paste, and xanthan gum and process on high speed for 1 minute until smooth.
Pour into tall shake glasses, sprinkle with chocolate shavings, and serve immediately.

Nutrition:
Calories: 190
Fat: 4.1g
Fiber:1.1 g
Carbohydrates:0.5 g
Protein: 2g

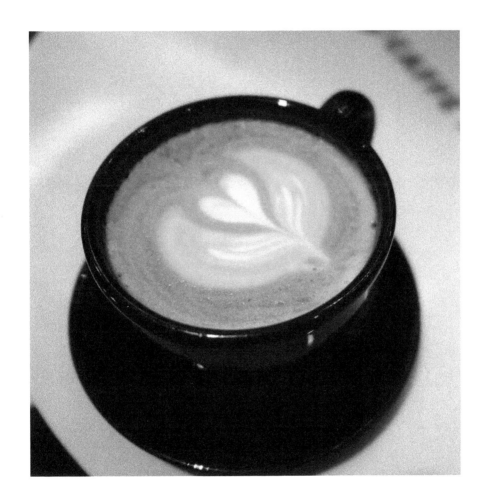

CPSIA information can be obtained
at www.ICGtesting.com
Printed in the USA
BVHW061035220321
603178BV00004B/264